Bedside Manner 101

Hanan Waite, RN, BSN

Bedside Manner 101

Copyright © 2013 Hanan Waite

ISBN 978-1-300-61737-2

Standard licensed material

Published by Lulu Press, Inc January, 2013

For my son, Ramzi

A special thanks to all the patients I have cared for.

This book was inspired by all of you.

Thanks to my sister Tina for motivating me always to put my

thoughts on paper.

Foreword

I am not a professional writer. I have never before written a book. I put together this book with all of the aspects of bedside manner that I feel are crucial to a workplace that involves caring for people. The experiences are through the eyes of a registered nurse and a mother.

Table of Contents

Chapter 1

My Story

I had my son by emergency Cesarean section on February 19th, 2011. He came 10 weeks prematurely, it was much too early. I was off that Saturday, the day that I had my son. Because I had only felt one kick from the baby all day, I checked into the labor and delivery unit at the hospital where I worked as a post-partum, mother-baby RN. My son had been a laid back baby throughout the pregnancy, but today, he was exceptionally quiet. It was around 3pm and I had not felt a single kick all day. As you can imagine, this drove me insane! I drove to the hospital, knowing in the back of my mind, that something was wrong; a thirty minute drive I made on my own because my husband was at work. I simply sent him a message via text before I left my house, to let him know that I was on my way to the hospital to check things out, and make sure that the baby was doing okay. He said "okay, don't worry baby, everything is okay."

On my drive to the hospital, I called the doctor's office to let her know what my situation was. Because it was a Saturday, the answering service took a message, and informed me that the doctor on call would call me back. The doctor called me about 5 minutes later. After I told her what was going on, she asked me only a couple of questions and said, "it's probably nothing, but go ahead and come in to labor and delivery, and we'll check everything out." I explained that I was already driving in. She giggled.

I arrived in the lobby of the labor and delivery unit, and checked in. I was tense but kept telling myself that all was well, and not to worry. I got my paperwork at the admissions desk and soon escorted myself to my room; a triage room, small and simple in the back of the ward. I did not need to put on the gown that was laying on the bed, the nurse said. We'll call her Sara. She explained that I would probably be discharged shortly after she listened to the baby for a little while. She was overtly calm and I could tell she was thinking this was a routine procedure for a nervous, first time mother. She placed the transducer on my belly to listen to the baby, and right away, we heard a strong heartbeat. She said "we have a baby in there!" I was relieved! I recognized this nurse. I had attended the same nursing school with her a few years prior, but she was in the accelerated program, so she finished a lot sooner than I did. She did not recognize me, but I knew her face well. She would eat all sorts of strange snacks in class, and I used to enjoy watching her be so mesmerized by her own food. She was one of those people that made you hungry when you watch them eat. She was just as cold to me as she was in class. Pleasant, but no bedside manner. She reminded me of Lucy Lui in Ally Mcbeal. In that show, she never smiled, and when asked why, she said she didn't want to get wrinkles. That thought made me smile...the only time I did for the next several hours.

Sara said to me, "just rest, we'll listen to the baby for a while, and then send you home if all goes well." She left the room. After about 30 minutes, she came back into my room to let me know that she had not seen any variability in the fetus, meaning his heart rate was not following a healthy up and down rate that is to be expected at this gestational age. She explained, however, that it did go down for a second at one point. In a healthy fetus, there needs to be accelerations and decelerations in the heart rate. My baby had one deceleration without an acceleration. My anxiety level heightened. She said, "let's take your blood pressure." At this point, she had not yet taken any vital signs. It was 154/104! She says, "you have high blood pressure!" In my mind, all I could think was really? Why did you not check my vital signs when I first came in?

Sara explains that she would have to let the obstetrician be aware of how high my blood pressure was, and also because my baby was not showing the proper reactivity. Soon after she told me that, she quickly comes back into my room and lets me know that the doctor has ordered fluids to be hung, and that she had put some dextrose in the bag to see if the baby would react to it. A healthy fetus usually reacts well to dextrose and begins to move around. Right then, I had a gut feeling that things were about to take a turn for the worse.

The attending doctor came in soon after the fluids were hung. She was the same one I had spoken to on the phone. We'll call her Dr. Deed. She was lovely. I was acquainted with her just because she was one of the obstetricians on the floor I worked on. We had spoken briefly before, and she had actually given me some advice once about my pregnancy, but I had never seen her during one of my routine doctor visits. She was very professional, and explained to me the pros and cons of having a premature baby at only 30 weeks gestation. She explained that she was not certain that

I was about to have the baby that day, but she still needed to inform me of all the possibilities just in case I did. She explained about brain bleeds that are common in premature babies, infection, and sepsis...thoughts that made my palms sweat even more, and my heart pound harder.

She went on to let me know that a perinatal doctor was on his way to perform an ultrasound; one that could really see what was going on with the baby. She said that in the mean time we had to get some lab work done and make sure that I did not have pregnancy induced hypertension (PIH). My blood pressures were rising higher and higher as I waited for the Perinatologist. My blood pressure went up as high as 160/110. I knew that my anxiety was not helping the increasing pressures, but I could not control it, which made me even more anxious.

The Perinatologist made it to my room in about 45 minutes, a tall, elegant middle-aged man. He was very professional, and had kind eyes. I felt comfortable with him, though I'd never met him before. He sat beside me and said "your baby has to wow me, because you have failed one out of 3 reasons to rule out PIH." PIH is diagnosed with 3 categories; protein in the urine, blood pressures of 150/90 or higher, and a fetus showing signs of distress. He placed the transducer on my belly, and within about one minute, he shook his head and said "this is much worse than Dr. Jones noted 2 weeks ago." What he was referring to was my visit just 2 weeks prior at the perinatal office.

(I went in for a routine ultrasound. All of the ultrasounds I had prior had been completely normal. This time however, the doctor noticed some "resistance in blood flow from the placenta to the baby." I had no idea what that meant but was a little embarrassed to ask. Because I am a nurse, the doctor assumed I would know what that meant, so he did not explain. Dr. Jones told me to come back in 2 days for a re-check in case there was just a mechanical error. When the technologist came in, she explained that this was related to PIH, and then I understood. I went home and researched for hours what this meant. The results scared me to death. I found that this resistance in blood flow was quite scary. It is a manifestation of PIH. Of course this scared me because of the possibility that the condition could worsen.) PIH is a potentially life threatening condition that women can get whilst pregnant. It is where blood pressures are elevated, and must be very closely monitored. It usually involves high blood pressure, protein in the urine, and swelling of the body.)

When he said that, I replied, "is this a good time to call my husband?" and he said "oh, yes!"

I did!

I was given an epidural, a urinary catheter, was shaved a prepped for surgery, and was whisked to the operating room all within 45 minutes of him saying those words. There must have been 10 people in the operating room. The lights were bright, the room smelled sterile...if there is such a smell, and my nerves were worsening the side effects of the epidural. I was shaking uncontrollably, so much so that I felt like my body was about to leap off the operating table. My teeth were chattering so hard, it seemed like they were about to break off.

After receiving my epidural, the team was eager to go ahead and start the surgery, but the medication had not completely numbed the lower half of my body. It was quite scary because the doctor and surgical assistant kept asking me if I could feel any sensation in the area that they were going to make the incision. It was evident how imminent they needed the surgery to be performed. The baby was struggling, and he needed to come out! That thought made me incredibly frightened.

The surgical assistant kept asking me "can you feel this?" putting the scalpel on my skin to see if I could feel it against my skin. Finally, after what seemed to be the 10th time they asked me, I heard the surgical assistant say "she's good." The room got really quiet after that, and I knew the surgery had began. Thank God, I didn't feel that initial slice, I was worried that I would.

I was suffering the effects of the narcotic in the epidural, and could not take a deep breath, which made me feel like I couldn't breathe at all. The anesthesiologist said that this was a normal side effect from the epidural. I could not take a deep breath no matter how hard I tried. I was sure that I was about to have a panic attack, so the anesthesiologist whispered to the nurse anesthetist, "give her some Valium." It did not seem to help. There was one very simple thing that calmed me down a little. The nurse anesthetist placed her hand under my chin and whispered in my ear, "you're gonna be fine, don't worry, just breathe." Her touch had such a calming effect. This certainly reaffirmed how very important human touch is, and how great its effects can be.

Needless to say, my husband made it to the operating room (OR) about 3 minutes before the doctor began incising. He was all gowned up in "OR" attire, and all I could see were his eyes through his blue mask and head cover-up. He sat by my side and held my hand during the entire procedure with fright in his eyes.

I was told that the only pain I would feel would be the tugging of the baby when they were pulling him out of the uterus. Well, that "tugging" felt like my soul was being ripped out of my body. It was the most physically painful experience of my life. I often compare it to the scene in the movie Braveheart, when Mel Gibson was on the slab at the end of the movie, having his guts cut out of him. Well, that is what it felt like; like my guts were being torn out of my abdomen. I later found out that with crash cesarean sections, that is quite normal. Suddenly, I heard someone say 20-0-0. I knew it meant that my son was out of the uterus at 8pm. I heard nothing, and my heart dropped. I was not sure what to think. All sorts of thoughts were going through my mind; "did he make it?" was just one of them. He was whisked away to the warmer. I was still not told anything, so I was incredibly stressed about his state and condition. My husband stayed by my side until he was asked by one of the nurses to come and take a look at the baby. He was petrified as to what our son would look like, being two and half months early. Still, he gave me a kiss and said, "I'll be back baby." I whispered, "yes, go and check on him baby." I knew our baby would be taken to the neonatal intensive care unit (NICU), being a 30 week old baby. I knew he would need oxygen, and possibly much more, so I was prepared for that, but I was definitely not prepared for the next 10 weeks that would follow.

The surgery lasted about twenty minutes, or so it seemed. Everyone was very quiet throughout most of the procedure. I asked the doctor if I could have sutures and steri strips (little band-aids) instead of staples. She said that because it was my first cesarean section that would be fine.

My husband came back to let me know how beautiful our son was. He told me how little he was, and that his hair was red...that made me smile. I had red hair until the age of 8 or so. I was orphaned at a young age, so with the curly, red hair, I was sometimes referred to as orphan Annie. After about 10 minutes of assessing my baby, the NICU team (there is a team of people from the NICU that come to the delivery room whenever there is any expected problem with the baby) brought him by my head so that I could see him for the first time. I was still being stitched up, and could barely see anything. I was straining to see him. All I could make out was that he was swaddled up tightly, with layers of blankets. I glared through the incubator, and finally was able to see about a centimeter of his forehead. My husband was told to accompany the NICU team, and escort the baby to the NICU on another floor.

I was taken to the recovery room shortly after the surgery. There, it felt like I had the shakes for hours. I was only there for half an hour. The neonatologist very kindly came down to show me a picture of my son, and give me a quick talk regarding his prognosis. That meant a great deal to me! She said that because I had received steroids prenatally, my angel's lungs were in good shape, and that she predicted he would be in the NICU for about 4-5 weeks. She brought me a picture of him that the NICU team had just taken. I saw it, and was instantly happy. He was intubated right after delivery, which was incredibly hard to see, but most importantly, even though he was only two pounds and six ounces, he was perfectly formed and so handsome. All his organs were completely formed, he had ten fingers and ten toes, and his eyes were even open for the shot. I was so relieved. Just 30 minutes prior, I really thought there was a possibility that he would not make it, so even though he had been intubated, I knew he would be taken care of, grow strong, and come home. I was, after all in one of the best hospitals in the southeast United States of America.

After the recovery room, I was taken back to the labor and delivery unit for twenty four hours because I was put on Magnesium Sulfate, a medication to help prevent seizures when blood pressures are as high as mine were. I was told that I could not go up to the NICU and see my baby until I was off the Magnesium Sulfate. This was the most dreadful news I was given! I had to wait an additional twenty four hours before I could see my son? After what we had both just been through, all I wanted to do was see him, and hold him.

I was wheeled to my labor and delivery room, where I was to stay for the next twenty four hours. I was greeted by my nurse, whom I remember only because she very harshly massaged my fundus (the top of my uterus) really hard every time she checked my vaginal bleeding. Each time she did, it took my breath away.

As my pain escalated, one kind charge nurse randomly came into my room to check on me. She helped position me into a place that I could rest without feeling like I was being ripped into 2 pieces. The incision pain had started to kick in and it kept rising.

The nurse that took over for the 7 am shift the next morning was awful, and really the premier reason why I am writing this book. She came in my room and never assessed me. She wrote her name on the board only when I asked her who she was around 1130am. She was rude and paid no attention to me.

I asked to get up for the first time to clean myself up in the bathroom. It is preferred practice that several hours after surgery, the patient begins ambulating to prevent deep vein thrombosis, a condition that can occur with decreased circulation, and pooling of blood. She agreed. When I was getting up, she did not lend a hand in any way. The only thing she did was wheel the IV pole behind me. She just watched me do it all on my own. I was quite disappointed, but not so surprised because I was very aware that this is how some nurses treat their patients. In the bathroom, while sitting on the toilet, I asked her for a spray bottle to rinse myself off. She told me "oh, we don't have those here." She gave me some wipes to use. That upset me, because after twelve hours of bleeding in a bed, I was really looking forward to getting up and freshening up. When I got up from the toilet, my underwear fell to the floor, and she watched me as I bent over like an old, decrepit lady, to pick them up. It was so painful. I wished my husband had not left to the cafeteria just before all this began. I teared up. Maybe I was just being a product of my hormones, but I felt so sad and alone. That moment seemed to bring back some painful memories of my childhood, and suddenly, I felt tears coming down my cheeks.

The next nurse I had was not okay. She was pleasant, but I had to constantly prompt her about my progression. I had to ask to be weaned off my epidural and to have my urinary catheter removed. Still, she did not deny me any of my requests, so I have no complaints about her. She just had no bedside manner whatsoever.

Chapter 2

Meeting my angel

When I finally got to see my son, it was exactly 24 hours after surgery, and I made it to the the NICU with my husband wheeling me there. It was exhilarating, yet crushing at the same time. My son was so tiny, and so precious. He was in a humidified incubator, mimicking the uterus as much as possible. He was on continuous positive airway pressure (CPAP). He had been extubated (his ventilator had been removed), which was great news. I could barely see his face because the CPAP tubing covered it almost completely. I could only see his eyes. They were beautiful. He did not open them much at all, but when he did, it made me smile. His skin was so brand new and shiny, and almost transparent. I got to touch his tiny hand. He wasn't strong enough to grasp my finger. I was not allowed to hold him. All I could do was stare at him, and weep at his bedside. We stayed as long as we could, and then my husband wheeled me back to my room. I cried on and off all night that night. It was the toughest 24 hours of my life, but my

son was here, and he was safe!

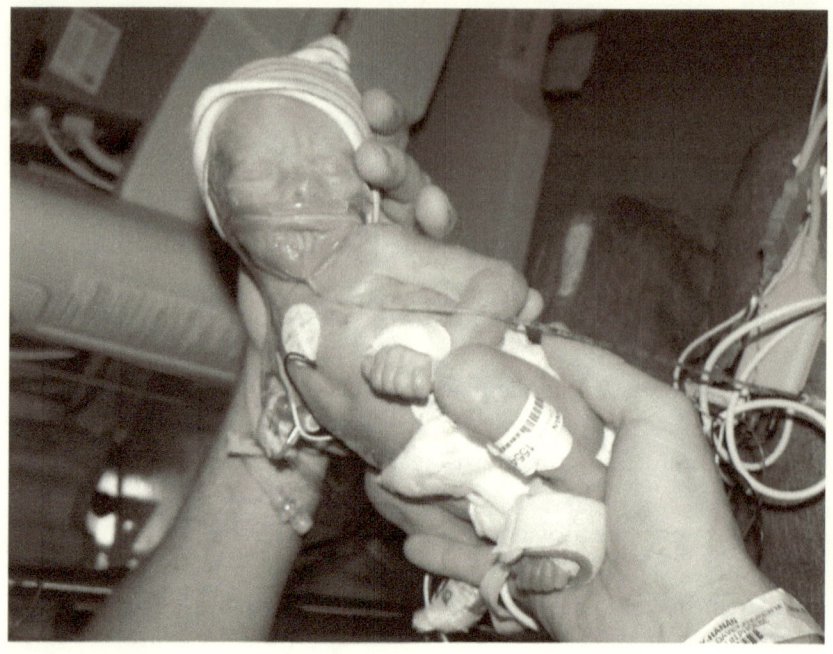

Image Above: My son at one week old in the Neonatal Intensive Care Unit

The next nine and a half weeks were tough. The neonatal intensive care unit (NICU) is often referred to as a roller coaster ride, and it is completely true!

The rest of the book is based on my experiences in the NICU. I have divided the stories into the Dos and Dont's of bedside manner based on my ten week experience in the hospital, as well as my experiences as a registered nurse.

Chapter 3

Bedside Manner 101

The Golden Rule: "Treat others as you want to be treated"

The Platinum Rule: "Treat others in the way they like to be treated"-Dr Tony Alessandra

In health care, we used to abide by the Golden rule but we slowly realized that the Platinum rule is a smarter, more customer friendly approach to service excellence. I believe that in taking care of fellow human beings, there are benefits to both these rules. For the majority of the time, it is far more important to treat others as they would want to be treated, but there are exceptions. When introducing yourself to a patient, greet them the way you would want to be greeted; a genuine smile, and eye contact. After you have established rapport, then you will be better able to treat him/her how they would like. Until then, you have no idea, so you treat them as kindly, sincerely, and as professionally as possible.

Simple Rules

Always knock on the door before entering a patient's room. If there is no door, you should still always ask if you can walk in. If there is a curtain, act like it takes the place of a door. Always ask if you can come in. Eg; "It's Nen, can I come in?"

When I was in the NICU, there was only a curtain giving me and my baby some privacy from the nurses, doctors, respiratory therapists, medical records personnel, house keepers, visitors, and others that were on the floor. For the first few weeks that we were in the NICU, we were on the critical care floor. My son's incubator was one of many that were lined up in his pod. What was quite disappointing was very often, a few of the nurses would sit at the desk behind me and chat about their assignments that they had during the previous shift, the baby shower they went to last week, or the vacation they took last month...all whilst I would be sitting directly in front of them, sobbing and talking to my infant in his incubator. I have never before felt so invisible. That was by far one

of the hardest aspects of being in the NICU, constantly being
unnoticed.

Always give eye contact when introducing yourself to your patient

When walking into a patient's room, it is important to
immediately give eye contact and introduce yourself as quickly as
possible. When you speak to someone without giving eye contact,
they tend to feel belittled and unimportant. It also negates any
attempts to establish rapport with the patient.

Always learn the patient's name. Some people like to be
called by their first name, others by sir/madam. Depending on the
patient population you are dealing with, you will have to learn to
read each individual and determine their wishes. There is also
nothing wrong with simply asking how he/she would like to be
addressed. I know that after working in the South, most of my
patients did not mind being referred to as sir/ma'am, but in
Southern California, a first name was just fine. You will have to
learn the culture and population you are dealing with.

Always show your patient that he/she is top priority even if you work in a high volume institution

When you are in a patient's room, try as much as possible to show them that they are your ONLY patient, your top priority. It can be hard when you are busy, especially in high volume institutions, however, it is crucial to treat each patient like they are special. During the time you spend with them, make it their special time, make them feel like they are your only focus whenever you are with them.

If it is a patient that requires some extra attention, it might take communicating to your team members to help you out; maybe even lend you a hand with your other patients and duties.

It may mean simply sitting beside the patient on a chair, just to listen to them, or holding their hand during a painful procedure or experience. It may only take up a few minutes of your time, just to make their day better. Some patients would love for you to pray with them. This does not mean you have to share the same faith, but be present, hold their hand, and be respectful!

Do not bring your own personal problems into work ie; do not have the issues that you are dealing with at home, displayed on your face

We all have personal problems, problems at home. Do not bring them into your patient's room; a sad, glum, disappointed face is the beginning of a rocky relationship between you and the patient. The energy that you enter a room with is probably the energy that will dictate how the relationship between you and your client commences and continues. How you start something is usually how you will finish it, so it is important to start the relationship on the right foot.

<u>ALWAYS</u>

- Knock on the door

- Say who you are; title, name

- Ask if you can enter the room

- Walk in with a smile

- Give eye contact

- Introduce yourself. State your title; "I am your nurse form 7am-7pm"

- Try to establish trust as soon as possible.

Do not assume that your patient trusts you

You never know who is behind that door when you knock. Do not ever assume that you can be a 'certain way' with all of your patients. Each patient is unique and has their own personality. It is up to you to figure out what it is that makes them comfortable, what makes them smile, and what makes them upset. There are some things that you may be able to say to one person and not to another. There may be things that make one person laugh and someone else cry or even get angry. It is your responsibility to read each patient to understand what kind of personality he/she has.

When you are given report from the previous shift about a "needy patient," do not go into the room with pre-conceived judgments about him/her

Many times during shift report, you are told a plethora of things about your patient other than their medical situation, usually the employee's opinion about the patient. Sometimes, it has to do with how difficult the patient's personality is.

Often times, there is a personality clash, and it is up to the medical professional to find out what the underlying problem is, and how they can try to fix it. Sometimes, the patient has trust issues from a previous experience, hence puts up emotional walls/barriers to protect themselves. Usually, with my experience, if you can read your patient, and treat them the way THEY want to be treated, they will progressively open up to you.

ALWAYS treat your patients the way they want to be treated! It works. When you treat anyone the way they want to be treated, not the way you would like to be treated, they usually respond in a positive manner. Caring for our patients like they are family is the easiest way to achieve service excellence every time. There will always be exceptions to the rule. Some patients would prefer you just do your job and leave them alone. You would still be professional, kind and gentle with him/her.

Helpful Hints

I repeat these rules again and again, because there have been countless times when I have witnessed the reverse occur. It saddens me to see patients disrespected and treated like they are a burden to the employee.

- Always knock on your patient's door before entering.

- Always introduce yourself upon the first time meeting your patient.

- Always give eye contact when speaking to your patient.

- Do not call the patient things like; cutie, sweetie, or any other unprofessional term

- Always offer to help your patient, even with small tasks.

- Most of the time, it is the simplest of things that make a huge difference to someone. When speaking with patients that were upset with the care they received during a previous experience, most of them explained that it was something very simple that set them off. Examples they gave me entailed some of the simplest issues.

Below are some of the common complaints that patients have. Most of them are repeated several times during a single visit.

"The nurse did not check on me when I asked her to. "

"I was given no eye contact by any of the staff here."

"She had an inappropriate tone of voice. She/he spoke to me like he/she was in a hurry."

" No one offered to help me even for simple tasks such as with latching the baby onto the breast."

"I could not reach my tray"

"I was in pain and no one cared"

The list goes on and on.

Because most of my experience comes from working with mothers and babies, a lot of the complaints and praises I have received about care provided, are from the mothers that I have taken care of. However, patients in all departments have similar complaints. Depending on how you look at it, the bedside manner given to a patient can make or break their outlook on their entire stay, and sometimes the hospital/organization as a whole. If you want a patient's view of their stay to be positive, then the care they receive needs to be accompanied by great bedside manner.

The mentality of healthcare staff that "we are saving the patients' lives, so they should be grateful!" is a very sad one. Some healthcare professionals think that because we are saving the lives of the patients in some circumstances, bedside manner is unnecessary, but this is very much untrue. In fact, all of the patients that I spoke with, were impacted more so by the bedside manner that they received over any of the technical, medical care they received. This does not mean that medical care is not important, but it is the smile on the surgeon's face, the kind words the lab technician used, and the touch the nurse gave, that the patient will remember. At the end of it all, we are all human, and it is basic human decency and interaction that makes the difference!

Bedside manner begins before you even get to work. Listen to music that makes you happy on the way to work, get in a good mood!

Be presentable! No one wants to be taken care of by someone that does not take care of themselves. Smile-smiles are contagious. Smile to your co-workers, maybe they will start smiling too! Smile to your patients-they will be happier if they see that you are happy.

Common Complaints from patients

- My nurse did not come when I pushed the call button

- No one checked on me until I called

- My food was cold when it arrived

- My food was not what I ordered (Muslims, Jews getting pork after specifically asking for no pork diet or vegetarians getting meat)

- No one told to me what was going on

- My nurse/doctor was mean/not happy/rude

- I was spoken to as if I didn't know anything

- The dressing on my wound/tape on iv's was removed without any compassion. That hurt!

- No one knocked on my door before entering

- I was treated like I was a number and not a person

- I often heard the staff gossiping about other patients/assignments

- The nurse/doctor introduced themselves or even mentioned his or her name

- No one cared if I was in pain

Start your shift...

Thinking about how your patients must feel.

Put yourselves in their shoes! This is such a common term, but seldom is it actually applied. Try to imagine how it must feel to be in the patients' shoes. Imagine, for most women, childbirth is the first and only time that they have ever been admitted to a hospital. Imagine how humbling an experience it must be for them to be dressed in a hospital gown-yes that is a very simple, but a strange thing for most people. Imagine how it must feel to have your vagina "checked" regularly in the labor and delivery unit. Imagine how it must feel to have some strange person conduct a vaginal exam on you. Imagine how it must feel to be told when and where everything is going to take place. Imagine being told how your day is going to go; a "care plan" is established for the patient, usually without his/her knowledge. This is to be expected, however, it is important to communicate with the patient what the plan of care is, so that the team is all on the same page.

"You are the first person who has ever taken out my IV this slowly."

Why should I have ever heard these words? Patients explaining to me that every other time someone has removed her IV catheter from her arm, it has been done roughly. Use an adhesive remover, alcohol, or peel the tape slowly before you pull the catheter out.

The same applies to the foley catheter, and all urinary catheters. I have found that when you ask the patient to take a deep breath and breath out whilst you pull out the catheter, that it is a much simpler, painless process than when you just yank it out.

"No one wiped me this way. The other lady just sprayed water on my vagina and used my dirty pad to wipe me down. "

That is despicable! How hard would it to be to get fresh wash cloths and wipe a patient down properly? Have you ever sat in blood for 12 hours? It feels disgusting! All you want is to get up, wash up, change your pad, and get a fresh gown. Most of all, you would like assistance from your nurse. But this is something a nurse's aide can do. It is not all just the nurse's duty.

If there is a writing board in the room, write your name and number down (if you have a cell phone or pager allocated), and make sure you tell the patient what the name and number represent. Most of the time, the patient has no idea what the name and number represents on the board. That should be one of the first things said to the patient upon entering their room. Introductions should be made with a smile and eye contact. "My name is Nen, I'm your nurse, and I'll be taking care of you today. I'll be here from 7am-7pm." This is very important. Several times, I would tell my patient what the number on the board was; my cell phone that they could call me on, and they were surprised. "I had no idea what that was on the board," they would say.

Make eye contact! I repeat that several times in the book, because it is crucial to forming a bond with your patient. It shows honesty and respect instantly.

Hold their hand when you can! My postpartum patient was hemorrhaging, so I had to transport her to another floor. I let my charge nurse know that I was leaving the floor with my patient so that she could watch my other patients while I was gone. She agreed. This patient was a very stoic individual, she had delivered twins naturally. Her pain tolerance was very high, but for the first time, I saw fear and pain in her eyes. Before she knew it, there were 4 other people in the room and the top of her uterus was being mashed down to try to stop her bleeding. She yelled out. I took her hand and looked in her eyes "you're gonna be alright," I said. She stared me deep in the eyes throughout the rest of her procedure. Later on that night, when she was stable, she called me into her room to thank me for staying with her during the entire procedure. She explained how terrified she was, and how important it was to her that I stayed with her throughout that experience.

Sometimes, the simplest act of kindness makes the largest impact. I have found through my short, yet condensed experience as a nurse, that it is the act of human kindness, above all, that makes a difference in people's lives and overall experience.

The nurses station

Sitting at the nurse's desk, reading magazines and chatting about celebrity gossip. A patient's husband comes up to ask a question about his wife and "Laura" the nurse does not leave her chair, but answers him from where she sits. She is surrounded by about 5 other staff members, and they all turn to look at the gentleman, who is now red in the face with embarrassment. Could she have been more impersonal? How hard would it have been for her to get up, leave the nurse's station, and address his questions and concerns in the patient's room, or even quietly in the hallway?

Is is maybe that sometimes we forget that the only reason that we have the careers and jobs that we do, is because of the patients that we care for!

In today's fast-paced, technological world, it is quite easy to put on the back burner, some of our true morals and values. Healthcare businesses have grown all over the nation, and yet, bedside manner is very much so lacking. The healthcare industry is full of caring, giving and humble individuals. Most people that choose this profession, do so with hopes of making differences in the lives of the people. Many aspects to the workplace can shape an individual's outlook on his/her career/job. In many cases, people find themselves working with several different types of personalities, various egos, certain negative individuals, people bringing their problems to work, and other issues that are detrimental to the best possible healthcare possible.

There are many definitions of bedside manner, but what I found, is that most of those definitions usually define the manner or conduct of a physician in the presence of a patient. **I believe that should also apply to everyone that comes in contact with a patient**. One may have great or poor bedside manner, whichever it may be, if you are working in the healthcare field, you have formed some sort of bedside manner. The goal of this book is to help reinforce good habits and have you be aware of the bad habits that I have noticed going unchecked at various institutions around the country.

I am writing this book in the hopes of improving the experiences that people face when confronted with the need for any sort of healthcare. One might be caring for patients today, and tomorrow might be in need of help themselves. Would that individual rather be treated in a friendly, caring manner by a real professional, or in an uncaring and disinterested manner by someone that seems like they would rather be someplace else?

Certain cultures have a more stoic approach to pain so they assume that their patients should need only need so much pain relief. A patient who had a cesarean section 8 hours ago had received one Percocet and one Motrin at 8am and nothing else for pain until about 3pm. Mind you the Percocet was 5mg and the Motrin was 600mg, which is not a substantial dose after major surgery such as a cesarean section. Can you imagine how this patient was feeling when I began my shift at 7pm?

She was angry, doubled over in pain, and didn't want to make eye contact with me. She was mortified. I knew that I had to change things around! I started my shift with an irate patient, but I was able, with much patience, to establish rapport and trust with her. Together, we were able to figure out her pain medication

schedule, which eventually made for a much happier, more pleasant young woman. The point in this case is that you can usually turn a situation around with little effort. Establishing rapport and trust should always be the priority for the healthcare worker.

Do not practice prejudice or pass judgment on certain populations

I was told a story about this 95 year old lady who was completely disrespected because the staff assumed that she was not lucid enough to understand or remember anything that happened in the hospital. This lady complained that certain staff members would come into her room to take and make their cell phone calls because they thought she was "out of it." Meanwhile, her granddaughter who was telling the story says her grandmother was, and is very sharp and completely aware. This poor lady was subject to being ignored, neglected, and even verbally abused. When she finally spoke up for herself, and asked the staff to leave her room to make their phone calls elsewhere, they simply told her to "shut up." Can you imagine how she felt? Utterly and completely disrespected! Thankfully, she was able to speak her mind after the event, and some changes were made. This kind of story is the horrifying truth to so many cases around the nation and around the world.

To discuss some of the horrific stories many have experienced would mean many more books. This one focuses only on bedside manner.

SERVICE EXCELLENCE

When talking about service excellence, you have to go ABOVE and BEYOND the expectations of the patient.

Some ways one can do this is;

- Provide not just what the patient needs, but exceed them.

- Provide outstanding care to the patient and their families.

- If there are any complaints concerning treatment or care, resolve them as soon as possible.

- Utilize supervisors whenever possible

- Respond to concerned patients as promptly as possible

- Make recommendations for improvement based on patient and family feedback

One of the great stories that I remember related to service excellence, involves a Portuguese-only speaking patient. She was rating her pain a 10/10. When I walked into the room, she was in tears, and immobilized on the bed due to pain. I used interpretation services to communicate with her verbally, but I did not need their assistance to know that she was in excruciating pain. She explained that her pain was not from the surgical incision, but from a severe migraine. She had received all the adequate pain medication, and there was nothing else that I could offer her at that time. Instead, I dimmed all the lights, turned on a meditation/light music channel, cooled the room down, and sat beside her on the bed. I massaged her head and neck, remembering all the pressure points that I could (I am not a massage therapist). I did not forget the pressure point located in the hand. She had been moaning from pain, but suddenly, after a couple of minutes, she was quiet.

As I listened carefully to her breathing, I noticed what seemed to be a snore. It was. She was asleep, and snoring. Amazing. After just a few minutes, I was able to exit the room, leaving behind a much more content patient. She then slept for a few hours. Her migraine was completely gone by the time she woke up.

You can only use the resources available to you. Not every institution will have a meditation or easy listening channel, or a light dimmer.

Use your imagination to come up with easy ways to non-pharmacologically take care of your patient's pain.

- Heat packs
- Warm wash cloths or blankets
- Ice packs
- Turning off or dimming the lights
- Sitting with the patient
- Massage
- Hair brushing/washing
- Grooming
- Meditation
- Guided imagery
- Distraction
- Simply ask the patient what might help or what has helped in the past if you are unable to come with an answer yourself

Sometimes, the simplest tasks make the greatest difference.

Specific to Doctors

Bedside manner can very much so affect the quality of care a patient receives, but it can also indirectly affect a patient's attitude toward their own care...their compliance, if you will. A patient is more likely to switch from a provider who has poor bedside manner to someone else who would listen to their suggestions and shows compassion and empathy. Approaching a patient with no empathy or sympathy has a tendency to intimidate or cause a patient fear.

A doctor with a poor bedside manner may actually cause a patient to perceive more pain, if the patient already has fear or anxiety. Having a great bedside manner, however, may help a patient care of themselves better, hence recover faster and better. This is not just limited to doctors and nurses, but to the entire team under the healthcare umbrella.

Doctors and healthcare professionals that are in the critical care departments tend to have a bad rap about their bedside manner. Surgeons, in particular, have a bad reputation regarding their way. Maybe it is the "I'm saving your life attitude." In my research, some people had great experiences with some doctors and others, dreadful. It was not just doctors that received these complaints, but since we are talking about them in particularly right now, we can focus on them.

A patient should feel comfortable telling you, as the physician, about private health matters and they should seek medical advice when they want to, without feeling as though they will be reprimanded, treated poorly, or disrespected in any way.

A good bedside manner should always include helping make the patient feel comfortable, allowing them the freedom to communicate with you, helping them out with medical advice and decisions, and showing empathy. You, as the doctor, should never come across as arrogant, abrupt, or rude.

The beauty about this topic is that a concern about beside manner has increased in the past few years. There are several schools for nurses and doctors who now offer courses on bedside manner and having an empathetic approach towards patients. Some hospitals make it one of their main focus points regarding their patient-doctor relationships.

I know that doctors have a heavy load. In the modern world, the patient load can be very stressful, but, just like the nurse, once in the patient's room, you should seem, to the patient like he/she is your only concern at the moment. They should have not one thought that you are in a hurry. You should not be curt or abrupt.

Be;

- Respectful

- Supportive

- Promote health as well as treat disease

- Communicate well

Always ask courteous questions, let people talk, and listen to them carefully. Try to always give unbiased medical advice. Let people participate actively in all decisions related to their own health care.

Evidence is a great tool, yes, but treat each case individually. Do not assume before walking in to meet a patient, that you can predict exactly who he/she will be or judge them. Help patients and their family members make the right decisions regarding their care via good, understandable education. Speak in terms your audience can understand.

Work cooperatively with other members of the healthcare team. Be advocates for your patients, regardless of who they are. Treat others the way they want to be treated. If you think you cannot abide by the platinum rule, then working in the healthcare field is probably not for you.

Simple steps for the doctor entering the patient's room

- Can you visualize the patient as being a member of your family? That would help tremendously with how you treat, view the patient.

- Of course, make eye contact, and try to establish rapport. Try getting to know the patient. Ask their name if you have not met them before. If you know it already, call them by their name.

- Listen to the patient, do not just talk at them.

- Ask the patient how their care has been; how they have been treated thus far. That will probably get him/her to open up to you. Ask; "how have the nurses taken care of you? How has the food been? How has your pain been handled?" etc

- Ask open ended questions. This will help you gain rapport with the patient and get more information about them.

- Try showing compassion and empathy.

Nurses in particular

Nurses, you already have so much to do every shift. I remember at my pinning service one of the speakers quoted someone that said "nurses are angels with sneakers on"...and it is very true!

- Of course the nurse should be well trained in whichever field that she chooses. Finding a specialty that she becomes an expert in, is a great way for that nurse to be happier with the career chosen. The more specialized she is in her field, the more knowledgeable she will be with her patients. This will help the growth of confidence in the nurse. Confidence is crucial in the nurse. Patients can tell when you know your stuff!

- Excellent communication skills-Nurses should have great listening and speaking skills. They should be completely comfortable speaking to a patient's concerns. They should know when it is time to listen and when it is appropriate to do the talking.

- A nurse should have excellent critical thinking skills. She should know the baselines of her patient and observe him/her so well that she would be able to identify when he or she is deteriorating. That takes great observation of your patient, which usually happens at the beginning of the shift.

- Nursing can be stressful and the hours are long. Try not to show it on your face and in the manner in which you treat your patients and coworkers. It takes dedication to continue the quality of care you promised to give when you became a nurse.

- Empathy and understanding are crucial for a nurse. It can be trying to be understanding when you have a patient who has a bad attitude because of what he/she is going through.

- Sometimes the nurse most of all, is chastised and verbally abused by the psychiatric, angry, alcoholic, belligerent patient. It is always very important to go up your chain of command and get security if the patient gets physical or if your ever feel threatened. However, if it's only a "bad attitude" then more often than not, you can most likely slowly gain trust through rapport and probably get a better attitude in return.

Those I spoke to mentioned these as qualities they would choose their healthcare professionals to embody

- Caring

- Empathetic

- Detail-oriented

- Adaptable

- Emotionally stable

- Critical thinker

- Hard working

- Loving

- Understanding

- Nonjudgmental/non prejudice

- Communicate well with others

- Treats others the way they want to be treated

- Responsible

- Positive

- Friendly

What patients listed specifically for doctors

- Respect

- Supportive

- Promote health

- Communicate

- Be courteous

- Be unbiased

- Treat your staff well

- Be an advocate for your patient

Finally, the most important point to this book is for all healthcare members to establish a good bedside manner; to treat everyone the way that person would like to be treated. From the lady in admissions who has you filling out paper work, to the secretaries, nursing assistants, nurses, and doctors. Everyone needs to be on the same team and that would make the workplace and the patient care much more exceptional.

About the Author

Hanan Aba El-Mahmoud Waite was born and raised in Ghana, West Africa. She lost both her parents at the tender age of 8, and was then raised by her maternal Grandmother. Life was anything but easy those days. However, she was fortunate enough to be able to come to the United States at age 15, and soon after, gained her American citizenship. For many years following, she struggled alone to care for herself, knowing that she wanted a better life than she had known in the past.

In 2008, after much perseverance, Hanan graduated from Georgia State University with a Bachelor's of Science in Nursing. In 2010, she was named by the March of Dimes "Nurse of the year-Rising Star," a great honor.

Hanan is married with a son. She still works as a registered nurse with mothers and infants. She founded a non-profit organization in 2012 called Earth's Angels, which is dedicated to eradicating maternal and infant mortality one mother and infant at a time. The organization will be working in impoverished areas to assist with basic medical supplies, clothing, infant feeding supplies, and much more. You can find out additional information at www.earthsangelsgive.org

"I am very proud to be a Registered Nurse. I take care of mothers and babies as if they were my own family."-Hanan Waite

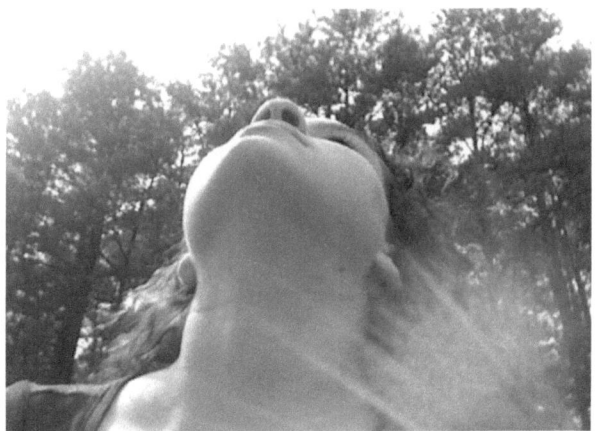